GIVE

YOUR BODY
A BREAK

Not a diet but a learning tool

Claudette Chayer

"Health is the greatest possession. Contentment is the greatest treasure. Confidence is the greatest friend. Non-being is the greatest joy."
- Lao Tzu

Table of content

Introduction

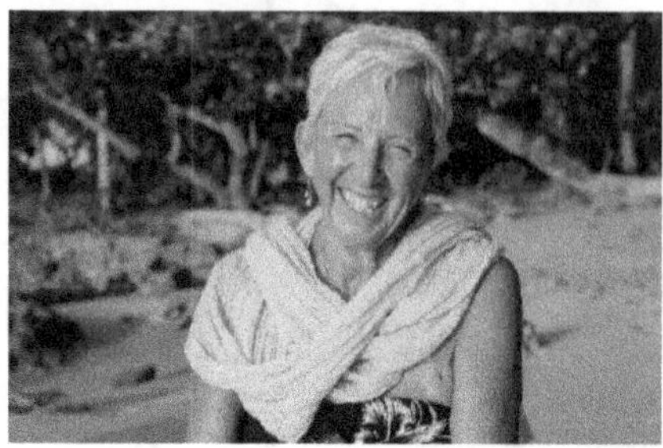

My name is Claudette Chayer, and at the age of 74, I continue to thrive in this wonderful world. I am free from illness and medication, thanks to my dedication to constantly improving my health through traditional and natural means. Surprisingly, I had never truly focused on the impact of food on my well-being, assuming that I ate well like everyone else.

However, in 2020, my life took a turn when the pandemic struck. Being in the Dominican Republic at the time, I often found myself avoiding looking at my reflection in a bathing suit, feeling disconnected from the image I saw. It was then that I realized I needed to lose weight and take action. That's when intermittent fasting entered my life. Intrigued, I decided to give it a try, and to my delight, it proved to be effective. In just six months, I shed 40 pounds of body fat that had burdened me for over two decades. Thanks to intermittent fasting, I was able to reclaim the weight I had in my twenties!

To achieve this, I chose to fast for 16 hours each day, enjoying a fruit-based lunch and a regular meal at dinner time. I discovered that I could be healthy without being too strict with myself. While I still indulged in occasional treats like wine and chocolate, I focused on consuming ample vegetables, cutting out sugar, and reducing my meat intake. This approach allowed me to maintain my weight, but I still experienced joint pain, liver issues, and struggled with sleep while occasionally gaining a few pounds.

That's when I stumbled upon a program that offered insights into the impact of food on our bodies. Intrigued, I embarked on a 90-day challenge, following a keto diet, eager to learn more. This experience provided valuable knowledge about my body and how it reacts to certain foods. I discovered that some seemingly healthy foods were actually causing inflammation within me. By eliminating those foods, I not only reduced inflammation but also continued to lose weight. I have since made healthier choices and significantly improved my overall health and well-being. I am now pain-free and full of vibrant energy. The best part is that I have been able to maintain my weight while feeling absolutely fantastic.

It has been three years since I embarked on this journey, and I still feel incredible. I am proud of my physique, as it reflects my dedication to a healthy lifestyle. I both look and feel great, thoroughly appreciating every precious moment of my life.

My findings

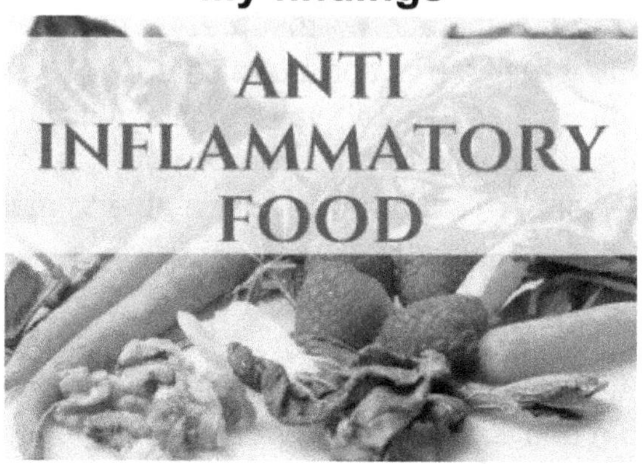

I discovered something quite surprising: inflammation, which occurs when our bodies try to heal from injury or infection, can be caused by various factors. Stress, lack of sleep, and most notably, certain foods can trigger inflammation. If we consume excessive amounts of these "bad" foods, we may experience chronic inflammation, leading to serious health issues like joint pain, digestive problems, heart disease, and even cancer.

Some of the most common culprits behind inflammation include sugar, processed foods, red meat, fried food, dairy products, and foods high in refined carbs. These items can disrupt our blood sugar levels and promote the growth of harmful gut bacteria, exacerbating inflammation. By reducing our consumption of these foods, we may experience improved well-being, better digestion, and overall better health.

In addition to eliminating inflammatory foods, it's crucial to incorporate anti-inflammatory foods into our diets. Leafy greens, berries, fatty fish, nuts, and whole grains are excellent choices as they are rich in antioxidants, vitamins, and minerals that can help reduce inflammation and support overall health.

While it may seem challenging to change our eating habits, there are a few reasons why it can be tough. We may have been accustomed to a certain way of eating for a long time, making it difficult to switch gears. Sometimes, stress can lead us to crave unhealthy foods. Additionally, it might be challenging to identify which foods are best for us or find them readily available. However, with persistence and motivation, we can make these changes. Seeking support from others is also perfectly acceptable. By making healthier choices and embracing a more nutritious diet, we will experience improved well-being.

It's essential to shift our perspective on food and view it as fuel for our bodies rather than a source of comfort or pleasure. Prioritizing nutrient-dense foods that provide energy and promote overall health, such as vegetables, fruits, lean proteins, and healthy fats, is key. Strict and restrictive diets can often backfire and reinforce negative behaviors, so finding a balanced approach that works for each individual is crucial.

It's natural to worry that we might have to give up the foods we enjoy or that the journey will be too difficult or confusing. However, by persisting and making gradual changes to our diet, we will begin to feel better. Our aches and pains may diminish, and our energy levels will increase, resulting in a sense of pride and accomplishment.

In this book, I will share the valuable information I have researched and the personal experiences I have gained on my journey, with the hope that it will serve as a guiding light for you as you embark on your own path of transforming your food habits. Often, we find ourselves trapped in habits that we are not even aware of their origins. However, it is important to recognize that habits can be changed through knowledge and conscious effort.

It is often said that it takes 21 days to change a habit, which may seem like a daunting task at first. However, when we consider the long-term benefits and the positive impact it can have on our health and well-being, 21 days is a relatively short period of time. By committing to this process of change, you have the power to reshape your relationship with food and unlock a healthier, happier version of yourself.

Throughout this book, you will find practical advice, actionable steps, and insightful tips that will empower you to make informed choices about your diet. I will share evidence-based research on the effects of certain foods, the benefits of incorporating anti-inflammatory options, and how to navigate the challenges that may arise during this transformative journey.

Remember, change is not always easy, and you may encounter obstacles along the way. But with patience, persistence, and a willingness to learn and adapt, you can overcome these hurdles and create lasting positive change in your life. Together, we will explore the power of knowledge and how it can empower you to make healthier choices, one day at a time.

So, let's embark on this journey together, armed with the knowledge and determination to transform our food habits and embrace a healthier and more fulfilling lifestyle. With each passing day, you will grow stronger, wiser, and closer to achieving the vibrant health and well-being you deserve.

.

It is time to make a change

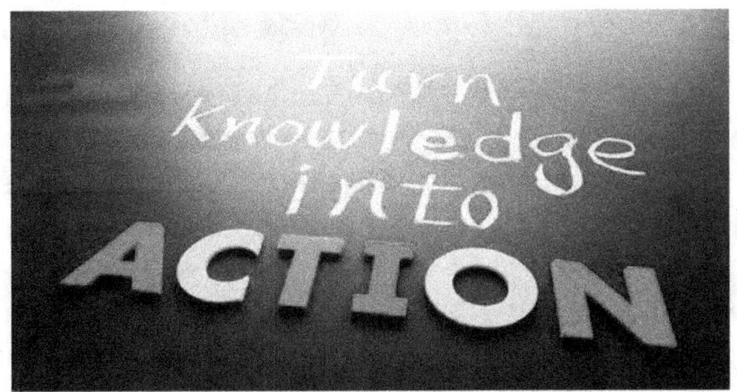

Our world is inundated with conflicting messages about what we should and shouldn't eat, making it challenging to navigate through the sea of nutrition advice. It's no wonder we feel confused and overwhelmed when faced with conflicting recommendations. The government food plan may endorse milk and meat, while vegans advocate avoiding them. With various diets like Mediterranean, keto, plant-based, and carnivore gaining popularity, it's difficult to determine which one is the best choice for our health.

In the midst of this confusion, one thing remains clear: we must take ownership of our health and well-being by educating ourselves about food and nutrition. This means conducting our own research, seeking guidance from qualified experts such as nutritionists and dietitians, and tuning in to our own bodies' signals.

The key is to adopt a balanced, informed, and individualized approach to our eating habits. By doing so, we can nourish our bodies and minds, establish healthy relationships with food, and live our best and healthiest lives.

It is crucial to note that taking control of our health means being mindful of what we eat. By paying attention to how different foods affect our bodies, we can identify those that may not agree with us and those that can potentially cause harm.

While some may perceive healthy eating as boring or restrictive, I want to dispel that myth. Countless nutritious and delicious recipes are available that cater to a variety of taste preferences. Cooking and exploring new flavors can be an enjoyable and fulfilling experience. Let's embark on this culinary adventure, discovering mouthwatering dishes that not only satisfy our cravings but also nourish our bodies.

As we journey through life, let us cultivate an open-minded attitude. This entails being willing to listen to different perspectives and ideas, even if they challenge our own beliefs. When it comes to changing our eating habits, it is important to focus on the opportunities for growth and learning rather than solely on the perceived difficulties. By approaching new ideas with an open mind and heart, we can expand our knowledge and experience personal and collective growth. So, let's embrace the invitation to view the world through open minds and hearts, embracing new possibilities on our path to optimal health.

Take a pause

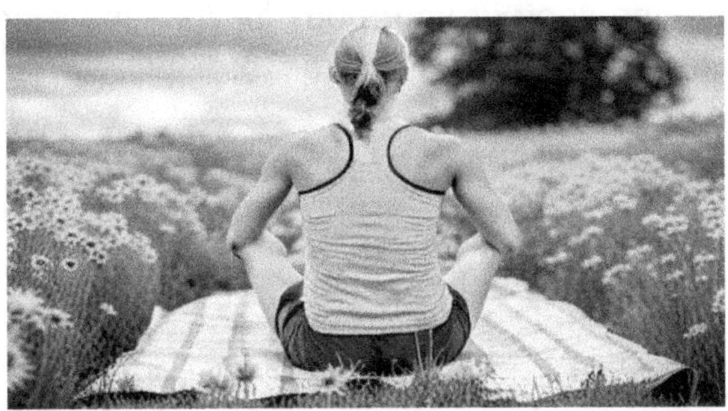

In today's fast-paced world, it's easy to become caught up in the whirlwind of daily life, often neglecting our own well-being. This can extend to our eating habits, where we may find ourselves rushing through meals, mindlessly consuming food, or even overindulging due to stress or other factors.

Taking a pause from eating can serve as a valuable opportunity to reset and reevaluate our food choices. Whether it's a single day or a week without certain foods, or simply incorporating breaks between meals, this pause allows us to focus on listening to our bodies, practicing mindfulness in our eating patterns, and consciously selecting the nourishment we provide ourselves. By doing so, we grant ourselves a well-deserved rest, enabling us to reflect on our food choices and potentially make healthier decisions moving forward.

There are numerous ways to approach a pause from eating, and it's important to find what works best for us as individuals. Some may find benefit in a cleanse or detox, while others may opt to eliminate specific types of food for a designated period. Alternatively, practicing mindful eating can involve savoring each bite, paying attention to the physical sensations experienced during meals.

Ultimately, taking a pause from eating can be a powerful tool in our journey towards cultivating a healthier relationship with food. By becoming more intentional about what and when we eat, we develop a deeper appreciation for the role food plays in our lives and become more attuned to our bodies' needs. So, whenever you feel that you may have overindulged or your body is signaling a need for a break, it's important to listen and respond accordingly.

Here are some suggestions:

Intermittent Fasting:

Giving our bodies a break from food for certain hours or days can promote a process called autophagy. Autophagy is a natural cellular mechanism that involves breaking down and recycling old or damaged parts of cells and organelles. It plays a critical role in maintaining cellular health, promoting longevity, and supporting cellular stress responses.

Intermittent fasting, which involves periods of fasting and eating, has been reported to have numerous health benefits. These benefits may include weight loss, improved heart health, reduced inflammation, enhanced brain function, and a decreased risk of chronic diseases such as diabetes, cancer, and Alzheimer's Some studies have even suggested that intermittent fasting may support healthy aging and increase lifespan However, it's important to note that individual results may vary, and it's always advisable to consult with a healthcare professional before starting any new diet or fasting routine.

By incorporating periods of fasting or giving our bodies a break from certain foods, we can potentially activate autophagy and support our cellular health. This process allows our cells to clear out and recycle damaged components, promoting overall cellular efficiency and well-being.

It's worth mentioning that autophagy is just one aspect of our body's complex systems, and it's important to adopt a holistic approach to our health. This includes maintaining a balanced diet, engaging in regular physical activity, managing stress, and getting adequate sleep. By taking a comprehensive approach to our well-being, we can optimize our health and support our bodies in functioning at their best.

Remember, while the concept of autophagy and intermittent fasting may hold potential benefits, it's essential to listen to our bodies and prioritize our overall health and well-being. Each person is unique, and it's important to find an approach to eating and fasting that works best for our individual needs and lifestyle.

There are several different ways of practicing intermittent fasting. Here are some of the most popular methods:

Method 16/8

This involves fasting for 16 hours per day and restricting your eating to an 8-hour window.

Method OMAD
This stands for One Meal A Day, where you fast for 23 hours and have one large meal within a one-hour eating window.

Method Alternate-day fasting
This involves alternating between days of normal eating and days of calorie restriction or fasting.

Method 5:2

This involves consuming a normal diet for 5 days and fasting for 2 non-consecutive days.

It is a common myth that we must eat three meals a day to stay healthy. However, the truth is that skipping one or many meals can be entirely safe and even beneficial for our bodies. When we do not eat, our body taps into its stored reserves and can retrieve all the necessary nutrients for proper functioning from our fat stores.

There are several normal reactions that the body may exhibit when eliminating toxins. One example is the Herxheimer reaction, which is a temporary worsening of symptoms that can occur when the body is eliminating toxins faster than it can handle. Other reactions may include digestive issues like diarrhea or constipation, headaches or migraines, fatigue, body aches, joint pains, or skin rashes. It's important to note that the body is designed to naturally detoxify itself, and not everyone will experience these symptoms.

However, it's crucial to remember that if you are experiencing health issues, it's important to consult with a healthcare provider before starting any new diet or fasting routine. They can provide personalized guidance and ensure that any changes you make align with your specific health needs and goals.

Juicing:

Juicing has gained popularity as a means to increase nutrient intake and support overall health. It involves extracting juice from fruits and vegetables using a juicing machine, resulting in a concentrated source of vitamins, minerals, and antioxidants.

One of the primary benefits of juicing is the convenience and ease of accessing a variety of nutrients in one glass. For individuals who struggle to consume enough fruits and vegetables, juicing provides a simpler way to obtain these key nutrients. Additionally, juicing allows for the consumption of a broader range of produce, including those that may be less appealing in their whole form.

Another advantage of juicing is the potential to enhance nutrient absorption. By removing the fiber during the juicing process, the nutrients become more readily absorbed into the bloodstream. This can be particularly beneficial for individuals with digestive issues that may hinder nutrient absorption from whole foods.

Furthermore, juicing can contribute to immune system support. The vitamins, minerals, and antioxidants found in fresh juice can bolster immune function, helping to defend against illness and disease. Certain fruits and vegetables, such as oranges and carrots, are especially rich in immune-boosting nutrients like vitamin C and beta-carotene.

Additionally, juicing can help alleviate hunger. Since there are no restrictions on the quantity consumed, one can drink juice throughout the day to satisfy hunger.

In summary, juicing offers a convenient and nutrient-dense approach to increasing fruit and vegetable intake, improving nutrient absorption, and supporting immune function. However, it's important to note that fluid intake should not rely solely on juicing. Adequate hydration is crucial for overall health, and it's recommended to consume at least 8 cups of water or other fluids daily.

It's worth mentioning that sugary drinks and excessive alcohol consumption can have negative effects on digestion. Therefore, it is advisable to opt for healthy, non-sugary beverages like water, herbal tea, or fresh juice to aid digestion.

As with any dietary approach, it's essential to consult with a healthcare professional before starting a juicing regimen, especially for individuals with underlying health conditions.

Eating raw foods:

Consuming only light or raw foods such as salads, fruits, or vegetable soups can reduce the workload on your digestive system and give it a break. Consuming light or raw foods can provide several benefits to the body, such as:

- Increased nutrient intake: Raw fruits and vegetables are loaded with essential vitamins, minerals, and antioxidants that are beneficial for our overall health.
- Improved digestion: Consuming raw and light foods can aid digestion by promoting the growth of healthy gut bacteria, increasing fiber intake, and reducing inflammation.

- Increased energy: Raw and light foods are easier to digest, which means that the body requires less energy to break them down, leading to increased energy levels.
- Better weight management: Raw and light foods are usually lower in calories and fat, which can help with weight management, especially if consumed in moderation.
- Reduced risk of chronic diseases: Consuming a diet rich in raw and light foods has been associated with a lower risk of chronic diseases, such as diabetes, heart disease, and certain types of cancer.

You can also make smoothies out of vegetables using a simple blender. This allows you to retain the fiber and obtain a plethora of easily absorbable nutrients. It's just another way to incorporate a variety of nutritious vegetables into your diet.

It is always best to speak with a healthcare professional before making any significant changes to your diet.

Signs that your body needs it

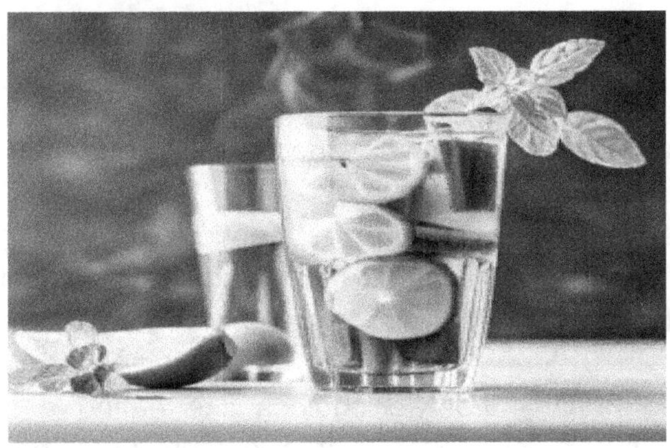

There are several signs that the body may need a break from food, including:

➤ Digestive issues: If you experience frequent bloating, constipation, diarrhea, or other digestive issues, it may be a sign that your body is having trouble digesting and processing certain foods.

➤ Indigestion and acid reflux: Frequent indigestion or acid reflux may be a sign that your body is struggling to digest food and needs a rest.

➤ Lack of appetite: If you find that you're not hungry, or your appetite has decreased, it could be a sign that your body needs a break from food.

➤ Chronic fatigue: If you feel constantly tired or lethargic, it may be a sign that your body is not getting the right nutrients or is overloaded with toxins.

> ➤ Headaches: Frequent headaches or migraines can be a sign that your body is struggling to break down and process food, and needs a break.

> ➤ Even skin problems: Skin issues such as acne, eczema, or rashes may be a sign of sensitivity or allergy to certain foods or ingredients.

> ➤ And frequent illnesses: Frequent colds, flu, or other illnesses can be a sign of a weakened immune system.

If you experience any of the signs mentioned, it may be an indicator that your body needs a break from food. It's essential to recognize the symptoms and offer your body support in eliminating toxins.

By making healthy lifestyle choices like eating a balanced diet, staying hydrated, and exercising regularly, you can support your body's natural detoxifying processes and promote overall health and wellbeing. Remember, prioritizing self-care is a vital step towards a healthier lifestyle.

Remember that while pills may provide temporary relief by alleviating symptoms, they often fail to address the underlying root cause of the problem.

Focus on antioxidants in foods are:

- Vitamin A – present in carrot, sweet potato, raw parsley, egg yolk, liver, mango and tomato;
- Vitamin C – fruits and vegetables, especially citrus fruits (lemon, orange, grapefruit, tangerine, clementine), kiwi and strawberry;
- Vitamin E – present in oils (such as olive oil), vegetable creams, oil fruits (walnuts, almonds, peanuts) and seeds (sesame, sunflower, hemp);
- Carotenoids (pro-vitamin A) – are found in fruits and vegetables. Beta carotene, for example, is found in sweet

potatoes and yellow / orange vegetables (pumpkin, carrots, papaya, mango) and red fruits (blackberries, raspberries, strawberries);
- Polyphenols – present in a wide variety of foods such as vegetables and fruit, some along with carotenoids such as soy and derivatives, cocoa, red wine, teas and infusions (mainly green tea).
- And many more

Therefore, it is always advisable to speak with a healthcare provider before starting any supplement regimen to ensure that it is safe and appropriate for your specific needs

.

Why avoid certain foods

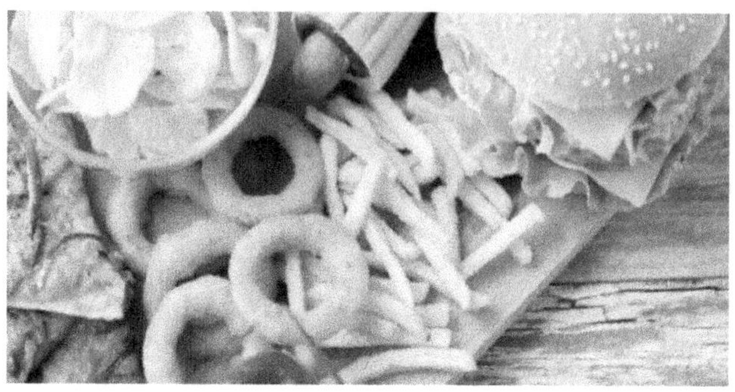

Food is a fundamental aspect of our lives, shaping our lifestyles, health, and overall well-being. It not only affects our physical state but also has a profound impact on our mental and emotional well-being. Our personal relationship with food is influenced by various factors such as our cultural background, family traditions, education, personal beliefs, and more.

Understanding and acknowledging these factors is crucial in comprehending the complexity of our relationship with food. It is important to recognize that there is no one-size-fits-all approach when it comes to food, and our approach should be tailored to our individual needs and preferences. Approaching the topic of food with empathy, mindfulness, and sensitivity is essential, considering its sensitivity from both cultural and personal perspectives.

From a young age, our mothers nourish us with the best intentions, associating food with love. As we grow older, we may develop emotional connections with certain foods, turning to them to fill voids in our lives or as a form of comfort.

However, it is becoming increasingly evident that the food industry has played a role in manipulating our choices by including certain ingredients in processed foods, leading to negative health outcomes. It is important to acknowledge that the production and marketing of these foods are often driven by big corporate interests that may not prioritize the well-being of the public.

Given these considerations, taking control over our eating habits becomes imperative. By becoming aware of the factors that influence our food choices and understanding the impact of processed and unhealthy foods on our health, we can make informed decisions about what we consume. Taking control empowers us to prioritize nourishing and wholesome foods that support our well-being.

Taking control over our eating habits enables us to establish a healthier relationship with food. It allows us to make choices that align with our personal values and goals, promoting physical health, mental clarity, and emotional balance. By being conscious of the foods we consume and the impact they have on our bodies, we can take proactive steps towards a healthier and more fulfilling life.

White sugar

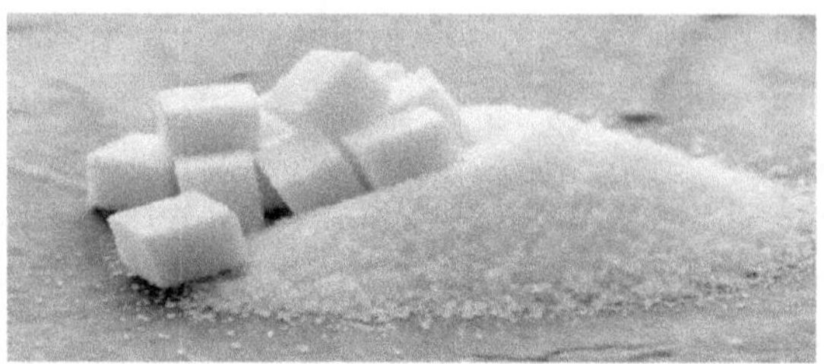

Sugar has a long and complex history that spans thousands of years. The cultivation and processing of sugar cane became a major industry in many parts of the world, and the demand for sugar grew rapidly in the West, particularly during the 18th and 19th centuries. However, the production of sugar was closely tied to the use of slave labor in many parts of the world, leading to widespread exploitation and abuse.

The food industry adds sugar to many processed foods for a variety of reasons.

> The main reason is that sugar is a cheap and effective way to enhance the taste and flavor of a product, making it more appealing to consumers.
> Sugar enhances the texture and mouthfeel of many foods, making them more enjoyable to eat.
> It acts as a preservative, helping to extend the shelf life of products and prevent spoilage.
> Consuming foods high in sugar can trigger an increase in appetite, leading to cravings and potentially overeating.

There is evidence to suggest that sugar can be addictive for some individuals, triggering a reward response in the brain and creating a cycle of cravings and consumption. This is because when we consume sugar, it activates the reward centers in the brain, releasing dopamine and other feel-good neurotransmitters. Over time, the brain may develop a tolerance to the effects of sugar, leading individuals to consume more sugar to achieve the same reward response.

Overconsumption

The overconsumption of sugary products has become a major public health concern. Excessive consumption of white sugar can have harmful effects on the body, including promoting obesity, liver disease, increasing the risk of diabetes, and certain types of cancer. Scientific studies over the past 15 years have increasingly highlighted the negative consequences of a diet high in sugar.

While sugar can provide a temporary boost to our mood and energy levels, in the long-term, a diet high in sugar can contribute to chronic health conditions and a lower quality of life. It is important to find healthier alternatives to sugary foods for a quick pick-me-up. Incorporating whole fruits or nuts into your diet can be a great way to satisfy cravings while providing essential nutrients. Making small changes like these can lead to significant improvements in your health and well-being.

There is also emerging research indicating a potential link between Alzheimer's disease and diabetes, often referred to as "Type 3 Diabetes." Insulin resistance and other metabolic changes associated with diabetes may contribute to the development of Alzheimer's disease.

Given the negative impact of excessive sugar consumption on our health, it is crucial for individuals to take control over their eating habits. By becoming aware of the factors that influence our food choices and understanding the consequences of consuming processed and unhealthy foods, we can make informed decisions about what we eat. Taking control empowers us to prioritize nourishing and wholesome foods, leading to better health outcomes.

Reading the labels

The consumption of foods high in sucrose, fructose, or glucose in excess can be harmful to human metabolism. It might surprise you to learn that sugar is often disguised by different names in the majority of food products. Reading the ingredient labels carefully is essential to avoid accidentally consuming sugary foods such as salad dressings, soups, bread, canned vegetables, biscuits for appetizers, and ready meals.

On the labels, the first ingredients are the ones that tell you the quantity in them.

There are many different names for sugar that can appear on food labels, including:

Agave nectar/syrup	Malt syrup/extract
Brown sugar	Cane sugar/juice
Coconut sugar	Raw sugar
Corn syrup	Dextrose
Molasses	Fructose
Fruit juice concentrate	High fructose corn syrup (HFCS)
Glucose	Sucrose
Inverted sugar	Lactose
Beet sugar	Maltose
Maple syrup	Honey

These are just a few examples, and there are many other names for sugar used on food labels. It's important to read labels carefully and be aware of the different names for sugar to make informed choices about your diet.

Avoiding processed foods and opting for home-cooked meals is generally recommended due to the significant amounts of added sugars found in many processed foods. Consuming excessive amounts of added sugars can have negative health impacts.

Cooking at home provides you with greater control over the ingredients that go into your meals. By **choosing whole, nutritious foods and limiting added sugars**, you can improve the nutritional value of your meals and support your overall health. Additionally, cooking at home can be a fun and rewarding way to connect with family and friends, as well as **explore new flavors and recipes**.

While it may not always be possible to cook every meal from scratch, **small changes** like **swapping processed snacks for fresh fruit** or **choosing whole grain options** instead of processed grains can have a significant impact on your health. By making **informed dietary choices** and **promoting sustainable food practices**, we can **help support a healthier and more sustainable world**.

Fruits

While fruits are an important source of vitamins, minerals, and fiber, they also contain naturally occurring sugars known as fructose. Consuming too much fructose, like consuming too much added sugar, can be harmful to your health. However, it's worth noting that the sugar in whole fruits is different from added sugars commonly found in processed foods and beverages. Additionally, fruits provide many other nutrients and health benefits that make them an important part of a balanced diet.

If you have a lot of weight to lose or you are diabetic, it's helpful to be mindful of the types and amounts of fruit you consume when trying to reduce your sugar intake. Choosing fruits with a lower glycemic index, such as berries, over those with a higher glycemic index, like bananas or grapes, can help manage blood sugar levels. Additionally, it's important to consider portion sizes when consuming fruit, especially for those with diabetes or prediabetes.

Overall, while fruits contain natural sugars, they offer many health benefits that should not be overlooked. By including a variety of fruits in your diet and being mindful of portion sizes, you can still enjoy the nutritional benefits of fruit while keeping your sugar consumption in check.

How to replace sugar

Fortunately, there are many ways to change the course of excessive sugar consumption and make healthier choices. One effective strategy is to avoid certain industrial foods that are often laden with added sugars and opt for homemade dishes instead. By preparing meals at home, you have greater control over the ingredients and can choose healthier alternatives.

Replacing white sugar with healthier and natural substitutes is another step towards reducing sugar intake. Options such as **maple syrup, dates, or honey** can add sweetness to your dishes while providing additional nutrients. It's important to note that while these alternatives are more natural, they should still be consumed in moderation as they also contain sugars.

When seeking sugar alternatives, it's essential to be cautious of **synthetic sweeteners** based on Stevia or Aspartame. While these may offer a calorie-free or low-calorie option, there is ongoing debate regarding their potential negative consequences for health. Consulting with a healthcare professional or registered dietitian can provide further guidance on the use of these sweeteners.

By making small changes and moderating your sugar intake, you can still enjoy sweet foods while maintaining a healthy diet. It's important to remember that reducing sugar consumption is a gradual process, and finding a balanced approach that works for you is key. As you make these changes, you can begin to appreciate the natural flavors of foods and discover new ways to enjoy sweetness in a healthier manner.

Retrain your taste buds

Reducing your reliance on unnecessary sweets is achievable with a little discipline and organization. By adopting these simple practices, you can create a balanced and healthy diet that supports your overall well-being.

Sugar has become a pervasive ingredient in our modern diets, and it can be challenging to reduce our intake due to its addictive nature. However, with determination and conscious effort, it is possible to retrain your taste buds and take control of your sugar consumption. Here's how you can accomplish this:

Gradual Reduction: Rather than attempting to eliminate sugar entirely overnight, start by gradually reducing your intake. This approach allows your taste buds to adjust more easily and helps prevent feelings of deprivation or cravings.

Prefer Whole Foods: Focus on consuming whole, unprocessed foods that are naturally low in sugar. Fresh fruits, vegetables, lean proteins, whole grains, and healthy fats should form the foundation of your diet. These foods provide essential nutrients and help satisfy your body's nutritional needs without the excessive sugar content found in many processed foods.

Experiment with Flavorful Alternatives: Explore natural alternatives to satisfy your sweet tooth. For example, you can use spices like cinnamon or vanilla to add sweetness to dishes without relying solely on sugar. Fresh fruits, such as berries or sliced apples, can also provide a natural sweetness to meals and snacks.

Be Mindful of Hidden Sugars: Be cautious of hidden sugars in beverages, condiments, and sauces. Sweetened drinks, including soda, fruit juices, and energy drinks, are often loaded with added sugars. Choose water, herbal teas, or unsweetened alternatives instead. Additionally, make your own sauces and dressings to control the sugar content and choose products with no added sugars whenever possible.

Give It Time: Retraining your taste buds takes time and patience. Initially, foods may taste less sweet, but as your taste buds adjust, you will start to appreciate the natural flavors of foods and notice the excessive sweetness in processed or sugary treats. Stick with it, and eventually, your cravings for sugary foods will diminish.

Retraining your taste buds and reducing sugar intake is a journey that requires commitment and perseverance. By gradually reducing your consumption, focusing on whole foods, and experimenting with natural alternatives, you can successfully break free from the grip of excessive sugar consumption. Remember, it takes time for your taste buds to adjust, so be patient and celebrate the progress you make along the way.

Soft drinks

Sugary drinks (also categorized as sugar-sweetened beverages or "soft" drinks) refer to any beverage with added sugar or other sweeteners (high fructose corn syrup, sucrose, fruit juice concentrates, and more). This includes soda, pop, cola, tonic, fruit punch, lemonade (and other "ades"), sweetened powdered drinks, as well as sports and energy drinks.

One can of a soft drink (354 ml) contains 33 grams of sugar, equivalent to **9.5 teaspoons** of sugar. This exceeds the recommended daily sugar allowance for the day, which is six teaspoons for women and nine for men, according to the American Heart Association. Continuously drinking fizzy drinks can lead to obesity, or at the very least, considerable expansion of the waistline.

We all know fizzy drinks aren't health tonics, but they affect the body in more ways that you may realize.
They do not give you any benefits.
They are empty calories.

Soft drinks have been linked to a variety of adverse health effects.
- ➢ Can lead to weight gain and obesity, particularly in children and adolescents.
- ➢ Increased risk of developing type 2 diabetes,

- Other health conditions such as heart disease and kidney disease.
- The acid present in soft drinks can erode tooth enamel and lead to tooth decay.
- Some research has also suggested that the phosphoric acid in soda may contribute to bone loss and osteoporosis over time.
- Those who consume more than 500ml of soft drink a day had significantly increased chances of asthma or chronic obstructive pulmonary disease.
- Drinking two or more soft drinks a week can nearly double your risk of developing pancreatic cancer
- People who drink on average one can of soft drink every day for 20 years have a 20 per cent higher risk of heart attack

Consuming large amounts of caffeine, which is present in many soft drinks, can have a number of adverse health effects.
- Potentially disrupting sleep patterns,
- High levels of caffeine can cause jitters, anxiety, and heart palpitations.
- May also contribute to high blood pressure and an increased risk of heart disease.
- May contribute to weight gain and other health issues over time.

It's important to moderate your consumption of caffeine and sugary drinks, and to focus on a balanced and healthy diet as part of an overall healthy lifestyle.

Alcohol

Alcohol in itself is not a sugar, and it does not transform directly into sugar in the body. However, alcohol does contain calories that can be converted to sugar by the liver, which then releases glucose into the bloodstream. When alcohol is consumed in moderation, this process is generally manageable for the body.

However, excessive alcohol consumption can lead to elevated blood sugar levels, which can be dangerous for people with diabetes or those at risk of developing diabetes. Additionally, heavy alcohol intake over time can lead to liver damage and reduced liver function, which can further affect the body's ability to manage blood sugar levels.

It's important to note that alcohol can contribute to weight gain and affect overall health. Alcohol contains calories, and regularly consuming alcoholic beverages can add significant calories to your diet. These additional calories can contribute to weight gain and increase the risk of obesity-related health issues.

Furthermore, alcohol can affect hormone regulation, including hormones that signal appetite, hunger, and stress. This can potentially lead to overeating or making poor food choices while under the influence of alcohol.

To maintain a healthy lifestyle, it's advisable to consume alcohol in moderation and be mindful of its potential impact on blood sugar levels, weight management, and overall health. If you have concerns about alcohol consumption and its effects on your body, it's always best to consult with a healthcare professional for personalized advice.

How to replace soft drinks

For those who love the fizzy taste, you could use soda water and add a sweetener in your drinks. There are a variety of alternatives to white sugar that can be used, including raw honey, pure maple syrup, and non-nutritive sweeteners like stevia or monk fruit extract. Some people also enjoy sweetening their drinks with slices of fresh fruit or a splash of fruit juice, which can add natural sweetness without the need for added sugars. Overall, the goal should be to find a balance that works for you and fits within a healthy, well-rounded diet.

Kombucha

Kombucha is a popular fermented tea drink that has gained popularity in recent years due to its potential health benefits. Kombucha is made by fermenting sweetened tea with a SCOBY (symbiotic culture of bacteria and yeast), which converts the sugar and caffeine into a variety of organic acids, enzymes, and probiotics.

Probiotics are beneficial bacteria that live in our gut and play an important role in digestion and overall health. Kombucha contains a variety of probiotic strains, such as Lactobacillus, Bifidobacterium, and Saccharomyces, which can help to support gut health and boost the immune system.

Kombucha is also a low-sugar alternative to soda and other sugary drinks, which can be a healthier option for those looking to reduce their sugar intake. The slight fizz and tangy taste of kombucha can be refreshing and satisfying, making it a popular choice for many.
However, it's important to note that store-bought kombucha can contain added sugars and other additives, so it's important to read the labels carefully and choose brands that use minimal ingredients and minimal processing.

Dairy products

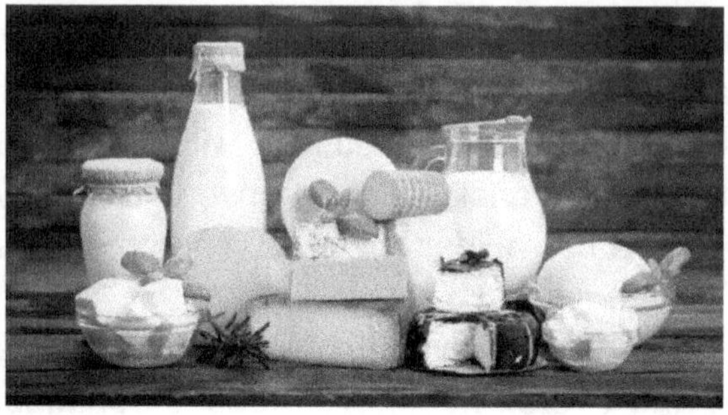

Dairy intake is a sensitive topic as we have been consistently told throughout our lives that it is crucial to consume milk for its calcium content. However, could we have been misinformed?

If we look at mammals in general, humans are the only ones that continue drinking milk after infancy. Initially, the ability to digest milk was limited to children as adults did not produce lactase, an enzyme necessary for digesting the lactose in milk. People therefore converted milk to curd, cheese, and other products to reduce the levels of lactose.

What's in there:
- ✓ Cow's milk contains water, protein, fat, carbohydrates, vitamins, and minerals. The exact composition of cow's milk can vary depending on factors such as the cow's diet and breed, as well as the processing techniques used to produce the milk. However, in general, cow's milk is a good source of nutrients, including calcium, vitamin D, and potassium.

- ✓ Pasteurization is a process in which milk is heated to a specific temperature for a set amount of time to kill harmful bacteria and pathogens that may be present in the milk. However, some people argue that the high heat used in pasteurization can also destroy beneficial enzymes and bacteria in milk, and may have negative effects on the nutritional quality of the milk

- ✓ Antibiotics. The levels of antibiotics in milk have increased, and in some regions, the authorized limit standards for antibiotics in milk have been raised. Antibiotics are used in cattle and dairy farming to prevent or treat bacterial infections. Some antibiotics can pass through the milk of dairy animals and can potentially cause negative effects on human health if the milk is consumed without proper testing and control.

- ✓ Hormones, including estrogen and progesterone, which are naturally present in the milk produced by dairy animals. However, the levels of these hormones can vary depending on factors such as the animal's age, reproductive status, and feed. Additionally, some dairy products may contain added hormones, such as recombinant bovine growth hormone (rbGH), which is a synthetic hormone given to cows to increase milk production.

- ✓ Did you know that it takes about 10 pounds (or about 4.5 kg) of cow or goat milk to produce 1 pound (or about 0.45 kg) of cheese, depending on the recipe.

Health issues

- ➢ Many research suggests that consuming casein, a protein found in milk and other dairy products, may contribute to joint inflammation in individuals with rheumatoid arthritis. This is because casein is a type of protein that can trigger an immune response in some people, leading to inflammation in the joints and other parts of the body.

- ➢ Symptoms of lactose intolerance can include vomiting, diarrhea, hives, and difficulty breathing, and in severe cases, it can lead to anaphylaxis, a life-threatening reaction.

- ➢ A systematic review conducted by Lu and colleagues suggested that increased whole milk consumption may contribute to higher prostate cancer mortality rate (2016). A recent study published in June 2022 found that men with higher intakes of dairy foods, especially milk, had a significantly higher risk of prostate cancer compared to men with lower intakes

> ➢ It has been shown that this food could be at the origin of many other types of cancer pancreas, colon, stomach, etc. It can provoke ulcers, chronic fatigue and diabetes.

> ➢ Excessive use of antibiotics can lead to the development of antibiotic-resistant bacteria, which can be harmful to human health.
> ➢ More and more people discover that they are lactose-intolerant

There has been significant lobbying by the dairy industry to promote the consumption of milk and other dairy products over the past several years. This lobbying has included efforts to influence national nutrition policies and to shape public perceptions of the health benefits of milk consumption.

However, there has been growing concern and skepticism in recent years regarding the health benefits of consuming dairy products, particularly in light of studies linking high dairy consumption to increased rates of certain health conditions, such as heart disease and certain types of cancer.

As a result, there has been increasing advocacy for alternative, plant-based milk options and a reduction in dairy consumption. This has led to some pushback from the dairy industry, which has sought to defend its products and maintain its market share.

Overall, the issue of milk consumption and the role of the dairy industry remains a debated and controversial topic, with various stakeholders advocating for different approaches to promoting health and sustainability.

It's true that the milk we drank as children, sourced from small farms with cows grazing in pastures, is vastly different from the milk produced by today's large-scale industries. In these industries, the conditions for cows can be less respectful, and cows may require medication to manage health issues.

This is a complex issue, and it's important to approach it with mindfulness and attention. While the use of medication can sometimes be necessary in ensuring animal welfare, there is a growing movement towards more sustainable and ethical approaches to farming. It's crucial to support practices that promote both animal welfare and ecological sustainability. In recent years, the dairy industry has undergone significant changes, prompting concerns related to environmental impact and animal welfare.

How to replace

It's worth noting that there are now numerous dairy alternatives on the market that offer sustainable and ethical options. These alternatives extend beyond just milk, with a wide range of non-dairy yogurt and cheese options available.

When it comes to choosing the right type of milk, whether dairy or non-dairy, there are a plethora of options to explore. Trying different types of milk can be an enjoyable experience, allowing you to discover the one that suits your taste preferences and dietary needs best. Different types of non-dairy milk are specifically suited for various uses, and selecting the appropriate kind can truly make a difference in recipes and beverages.

Source of calcium

There is a common myth surrounding calcium intake in dairy products and the availability of calcium in plant-based sources. While dairy products are often associated with being the primary source of calcium, it's important to note that calcium can be obtained from a variety of plant-based foods as well.

Plant-based sources of calcium include leafy green vegetables like kale, broccoli, and spinach, as well as legumes, tofu, almonds, sesame seeds, and fortified plant-based milk alternatives. These foods can provide significant amounts of calcium and can be incorporated into a balanced diet to meet calcium needs.

It's important to note that while dairy products are a good source of calcium, they are not the only source, and individuals who follow a vegan or lactose-free diet can still meet their calcium needs through plant-based sources.

There are many alternative sources that can provide this essential nutrient. Non-dairy milk options such as almond milk, soy milk, or oat milk are often fortified with calcium and can be a suitable replacement. Additionally, these alternatives offer a range of flavors and textures that can cater to individual preferences.

By exploring and incorporating dairy alternatives into our diets, we can address concerns related to environmental sustainability and animal welfare. These alternatives not only provide viable options for those with dietary restrictions or preferences but also contribute to a more diverse and inclusive food landscape. Whether it's through trying different types of non-dairy milk, yogurt, or cheese, embracing these alternatives allows us to make more conscious choices that align with our values while still enjoying the flavors and textures we love.

As consumers, we have the power to make informed choices about the products we consume. Choosing products from companies that prioritize animal welfare and sustainability can help promote a more responsible and sustainable approach to food production.

Cereals

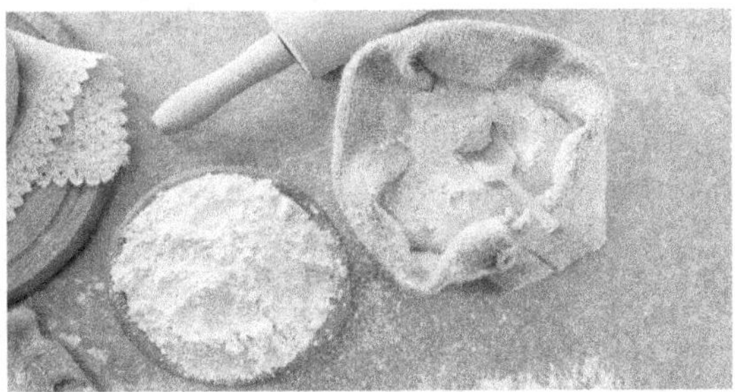

Another staple in daily food consumption is bread, and it can pose a challenge when deciding which type to include in our diet. The question arises: should we eat bread daily, and if so, which type?

Bread has been a dietary staple for centuries and can provide essential nutrients such as carbohydrates, fiber, and some B vitamins. Carbohydrates from bread are a valuable source of energy for our bodies. However, it's important to consider the quality and quantity of bread we consume.

When it comes to choosing bread, it's beneficial to opt for whole grain or whole wheat bread instead of refined white bread. Whole grain bread retains more of the natural nutrients and fiber found in the grain, making it a healthier choice. It's also advisable to check the ingredients list and ensure that the bread doesn't contain excessive amounts of added sugars or preservatives.

While bread can be a part of a healthy diet, portion control is key. It's important to be mindful of the amount of bread we consume, as excessive intake can contribute to weight gain and other health issues. The recommended serving size of bread can vary based on individual needs and dietary goals. Consulting with a healthcare professional or registered dietitian can provide personalized guidance on appropriate portion sizes.

Bread can be a part of a balanced diet, especially when opting for whole grain or whole wheat varieties. However, portion control and individual considerations should be taken into account. Consulting with a healthcare professional or registered dietitian can provide personalized advice on incorporating bread into a healthy eating plan.

Additionally, some grains may be heavily processed and stripped of important nutrients, which can make them less beneficial for overall health. For example, refined grains like white rice or white bread can be less nutritious because they lack the fiber and other important nutrients found in whole grains.

Gluten

Certain grains may not be recommended in certain situations because they may contain gluten, which can lead to health issues for those with gluten sensitivities or celiac disease.

> Gluten is a protein found in grains such as wheat, barley, and rye. It helps give structure to foods like bread and pasta by binding ingredients together.

> It is not uncommon to find these cereals in the composition of industrial products. Finally, nowadays, we are confronted with GMO experimentation, in particular on wheat.

> Furthermore, cereals contain trypsin inhibitors, which are compounds that interfere with protein digestion due to their ability to bind to and prevent the action of trypsin, an enzyme required for protein digestion. This can lead to reduced absorption of amino acids, which are important for brain health.

Health issues

- Gluten is known to cause an immune reaction in people with celiac disease or non-celiac gluten sensitivity, leading to digestive symptoms and other health issues including intestinal permeability, irritable bowel syndrome, inflammatory bowel diseases such as Crohn's disease.

- Cereals have a high glycemic index, which means they can cause a rapid rise in blood sugar levels after consumption. This has been linked to an increased risk of inflammation and insulin resistance, which can contribute to the development of a number of chronic conditions, including type 2 diabetes, obesity and heart disease. inflammatory rheumatism, acne or psoriasis, photosensitivity, eczema, hives, chronic fatigue syndrome, hepatitis and chronic pancreatitis, cancers, infectious and rheumatoid arthritis.

- Studies have suggested that there is a close link between cereals and certain neurological conditions such as migraines, depression, Alzheimer's disease

- Autism has been researched to be the consequence of deterioration and excessive absorption of peptides causing disruption of biochemical and neuro-regulatory processes. Finally, some studies have shown that a gluten-free and low-carbohydrate diet may help reduce symptoms of autism.

- One potential reason for these associations is the high concentration of pro-inflammatory compounds in cereals, such as gluten and lectins. These compounds can cause damage to the gut lining, leading to intestinal permeability or "leaky gut syndrome," which can contribute to chronic inflammation and a host of health issues.

How to replace

The best-known cereals for "gluten-free" are wild rice, quinoa, buckwheat and corn. Add to that coconut flour, almond flour, chickpea flour.

It can be challenging to replace wheat in our diets, as it's present in so many staple foods like bread, pasta, and many others. However, even if you aren't gluten intolerant or unsure if you are, it can be interesting to experiment with a wheat-free diet for a period of time.

There are many new products on the market that use rice and quinoa for pasta, which can be a great alternative. Additionally, there are numerous bread recipes available that can serve as a tasty substitute.

It's also worth noting that reducing your consumption of these wheat-heavy foods can also be a positive step forward. By incorporating more variety into your diet and exploring new foods, you may be surprised at how much you enjoy the change.

Meat and processed meats

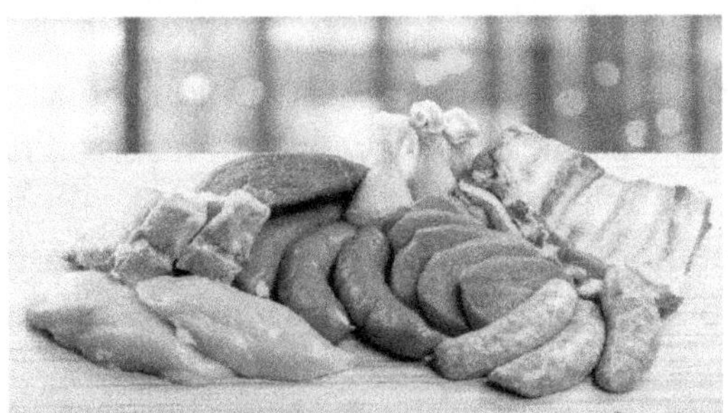

While meat can be a source of essential nutrients, excessive consumption, particularly of certain types of meat, has been associated with various health risks.

Health Risks

Here are some potential health problems associated with meat consumption:

> Cardiovascular Disease: High intake of red and processed meats has been linked to an increased risk of cardiovascular diseases, including heart disease and stroke. These meats are often high in saturated fats and cholesterol, which can contribute to the development of plaque in the arteries.

> Cancer: Consumption of processed meats, such as bacon, sausages, and hot dogs, has been classified as a Group 1 carcinogen by the World Health Organization (WHO). This means that there is sufficient evidence to suggest that processed meats can cause cancer, particularly colorectal cancer. Red meat has also been associated with an increased risk of certain types of cancer, including colorectal, pancreatic, and prostate cancer.

> Obesity and Weight Gain: High consumption of fatty meats can contribute to weight gain and obesity due to their high

calorie and fat content. Excessive calorie intake from meat, especially when combined with a sedentary lifestyle, can lead to weight gain.

➢ Type 2 Diabetes: Studies have shown that a high intake of processed and red meats is associated with an increased risk of developing type 2 diabetes. The high fat content and the presence of certain compounds in meat, such as heme iron and advanced glycation end products (AGEs), may contribute to insulin resistance and impaired glucose metabolism.

➢ Digestive Issues: Some individuals may experience digestive issues, such as constipation or an increased risk of diverticulitis, when consuming a diet high in red meat. These issues may be related to the low fiber content and high fat content of meat.

It's important to note that the risks associated with meat consumption can vary depending on the type of meat, cooking methods, and overall dietary patterns. Additionally, individual factors such as genetics, lifestyle, and overall diet quality also play a role in determining the impact of meat consumption on health.

How to replace

To replace meat in your diet, you can incorporate a variety of plant-based protein sources.
Here are some options:

✓ . Legumes such as beans, lentils, and chickpeas are excellent sources of protein. They can be used in soups, stews, salads, or made into burgers and patties.
✓ Tofu and Tempeh are soy-based products that are rich in protein. They can be marinated and used in stir-fries, curries, or grilled as a meat substitute.

✓ Seitan is a wheat gluten-based protein that has a meat-like texture. It can be used in dishes like stir-fries, sandwiches, or stews.

✓ Quinoa is a complete protein source and can be used as a base for salads, stir-fries, or as a substitute for rice.

✓ Almonds, walnuts, peanuts, chia seeds, and hemp seeds are all good sources of protein. They can be added to smoothies, salads, or used as toppings for dishes.

✓ Plant-Based Meat Alternatives: There are now many plant-based meat alternatives available in the market, made from ingredients like soy, peas, or mushrooms. These products mimic the taste and texture of meat and can be used in various recipes.

Vegetarian and Vegan Diets

Plant-based diets can provide an abundance of essential nutrients, including protein, vitamins, minerals, and fiber. Here are some key considerations for vegetarians and vegans:

✓ Protein: Plant-based protein sources include legumes (beans, lentils, chickpeas), tofu, tempeh, seitan, quinoa, nuts, and seeds. By incorporating a variety of these protein-rich foods into their diet, vegetarians and vegans can meet their protein needs.

✓ Vitamins and Minerals: Vegetarians and vegans should pay attention to obtaining adequate amounts of nutrients that are more commonly found in animal products, such as vitamin B12, iron, calcium, and zinc. These nutrients can be obtained through fortified foods or supplements. Additionally, consuming a variety of fruits, vegetables, whole grains, and plant-based sources of fats can help ensure a well-rounded intake of vitamins and minerals.

✓ Omega-3 Fatty Acids: Plant-based sources of omega-3 fatty acids include flaxseeds, chia seeds, hemp seeds, walnuts, and algae-based supplements. These can be included in the diet to meet the body's needs for these essential fats.

✓ Vitamin D: Vitamin D can be obtained through sunlight exposure and fortified foods. However, depending on factors such as geographic location and sun exposure, supplementation may be necessary for some individuals, including vegetarians and vegans.

✓ Balanced Diet: It's important for vegetarians and vegans to consume a varied and balanced diet that includes a wide range of plant-based foods to ensure they obtain all the necessary nutrients. This includes a variety of fruits, vegetables, whole grains, legumes, nuts, and seeds.

By following a well-planned vegetarian or vegan diet, individuals can meet their nutritional needs and maintain good health. It's recommended to consult with a healthcare professional or registered dietitian for personalized guidance and to ensure nutritional adequacy.

Reducetarian diet

Adopting a reducetarian approach, which involves reducing meat consumption and incorporating more plant-based foods into one's diet, can have several benefits for both personal health and the environment. It's important to note that being a reducetarian does not necessarily mean following a specific diet or eating pattern. It is a flexible approach that allows individuals to make choices that align with their personal preferences and values. Some reducetarians may choose to eat meat only on certain days of the week, while others may opt for smaller portions or choose plant-based alternatives more frequently.

Here are some reasons why being a reducetarian can be beneficial:

➢ Health Benefits: Reducing meat consumption and increasing the intake of plant-based foods can lead to improved overall health. Plant-based diets are often rich in fiber, vitamins, minerals, and antioxidants while being lower in saturated fats and cholesterol. This can help reduce the risk of chronic diseases such as heart disease, certain cancers, and obesity.

➢ Environmental Impact: Livestock production, particularly industrial-scale meat production, has a significant environmental impact. It contributes to deforestation, greenhouse gas emissions, water pollution, and depletion of natural resources. By reducing meat consumption, individuals can help mitigate these environmental issues and promote sustainability.

➢ Animal Welfare: Many people choose to reduce their meat consumption due to concerns about animal welfare. Industrial farming practices often involve crowded and stressful conditions for animals, which can lead to ethical concerns. By reducing meat consumption, individuals can support more humane and sustainable farming practices.

➢ Dietary Variety: Adopting a reducetarian approach encourages individuals to explore a wider range of plant-based foods, which can lead to a more diverse and nutritious diet. Incorporating a variety of fruits, vegetables, whole grains, legumes, nuts, and seeds can provide a wide array of flavors, textures, and nutrients.

➢ Cultural and Culinary Exploration: Reduce meat consumption allows individuals to explore different cuisines and cooking techniques that focus on plant-based ingredients. This opens up opportunities to discover new flavors, try innovative recipes, and expand culinary skills.

By embracing a reducetarian lifestyle, individuals can make a positive impact on their health, the environment, and animal welfare while still enjoying the occasional meat-based meal. It's a flexible approach that encourages gradual changes and allows individuals to find a balance that works for them.

Feeling overwhelmed

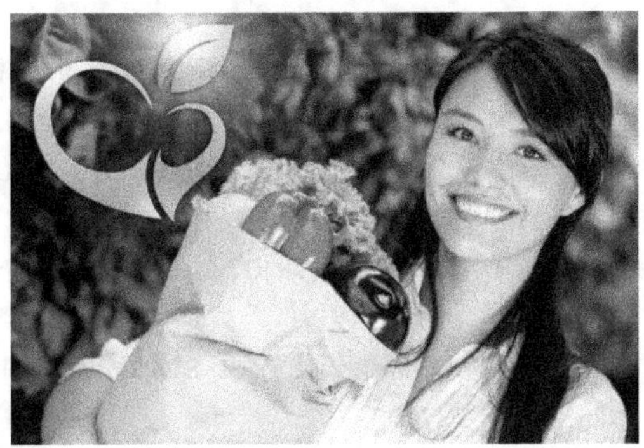

At first glance, all this new information about healthy eating can be overwhelming. But perhaps you already knew some of it and have already started making changes - good for you! However, we know that changing our eating habits is a long process that must be done slowly and at our own pace. If there's just one thing that struck you, consider starting there. Or, if you're in shock from learning all this, take a slow, deep breath and absorb the information gradually.

A good way to start would be to try incorporating some new recipes into your diet or experimenting with fasting or drinking more water. Remember, even small changes can make a difference. If you're committed to a long-term change, taking it one step at a time can help you achieve sustainable success.

Regarding lactose or gluten intolerance, the best way to determine if you are intolerant to these substances is to gradually eliminate the problematic food group from your diet and see if your symptoms improve. For example, if you suspect lactose intolerance, you can try avoiding dairy products for a period of time and observe if your digestive symptoms subside. Similarly, if you suspect gluten intolerance, you can eliminate gluten-containing foods and monitor any changes in your symptoms.

It's important to note that if you suspect you have a food intolerance or allergy, it's advisable to consult with a healthcare professional or registered dietitian for proper diagnosis and guidance. They can help you navigate your dietary choices and ensure you are meeting your nutritional needs while managing any intolerances or allergies.

Remember, making changes to your diet and lifestyle is a personal journey, and it's important to listen to your body and make choices that work best for you. Celebrate the progress you make along the way, no matter how small, and be patient with yourself as you embark on this path of healthier living.

Reducing sugar intake is a great first step towards improving your overall health.

- ✓ Making small changes, like swapping out white sugar for natural sweeteners like honey or maple syrup
- ✓ Replacing sugary drinks with soda water and a natural sweetener is another great way to cut back on sugar.
- ✓ If you enjoy fruit juices, try diluting them with water to limit your consumption of added sugars.
- ✓ Start reading labels and realize how many products contain sugar.
- ✓ It's also important to be mindful of timing when it comes to eating sweet treats. Waiting at least an hour after a meal before indulging in dessert can help you enjoy them in moderation without overloading on sugar.
- ✓ When it comes to natural sweeteners, options like honey and maple syrup can offer added health benefits while still satisfying your sweet tooth.

Remember, small changes can make a big difference when it comes to your health.

Journaling

The practice of journaling can help us become more aware of our food choices and any potential health effects. By keeping track of what and why we eat, we can gain a better understanding of our eating habits and identify patterns or triggers that may be impacting our health.

Journaling can also be a useful tool for identifying any food sensitivities or allergies we may have. By tracking our symptoms after consuming certain foods, we can pinpoint potential problem foods and make necessary changes to our diet.

Overall, journaling about food and its effects on the body can be a simple yet effective way to improve one's overall health and wellbeing. It encourages mindfulness and self-awareness, which can help us make more informed and intentional food choices.

Recipes

There are countless recipes waiting to be discovered and tried, making it an exciting adventure in the kitchen. Simply inputting the ingredients, you have on hand into a search engine like Google can uncover a myriad of possibilities, allowing you to explore new and delicious ways of eating. It's like a magic gateway to new culinary experiences!

If you're looking for recipes that are free from white sugar, dairy products, or gluten, there are several search terms you can use to refine your search results. Here are some suggestions:

For sugar-free recipes:
- "No sugar added recipes"
- "Recipes without white sugar"
- "Sugar-free dessert recipes"
- "Low carb sweets"

For dairy-free recipes:
- "Dairy-free cooking"
- "Recipes without milk"
- "Vegan recipes"
- "Non-dairy substitutes"

For gluten-free recipes:
- "Gluten-free cooking"
- "Recipes without wheat"
- "Celiac-friendly recipes"
- "Paleo recipes"

You can combine these terms with specific dish names, like "sugar-free chocolate cake recipe" or "dairy-free mac and cheese recipe", to get more relevant results. Additionally, be sure to check out cooking blogs or websites that specialize in specific dietary needs, as they may have a wider range of recipes to choose from. I hope these tips help you find the perfect recipe for your dietary requirements!

My main goal is not to provide specific recipes, but to show you how easy and fun it can be to change the way you eat, whether it's by avoiding white sugar, dairy products, or gluten. By using specific search terms, you can better refine your results and find recipes that meet your dietary needs. With a little bit of effort and creativity, you can transform your eating habits and improve your overall health and well-being.

Your body knows best

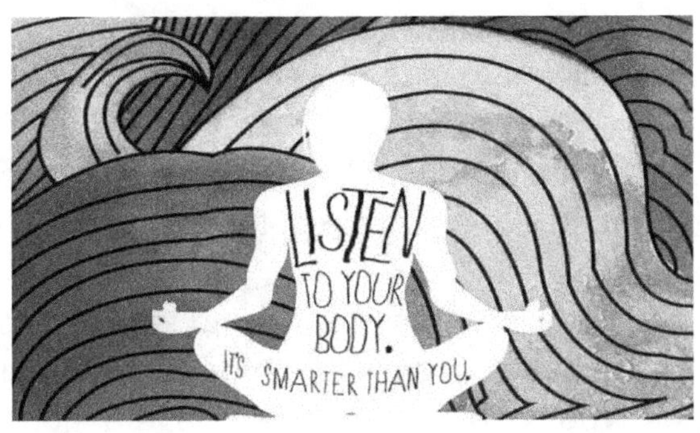

One of the most profound and transformative aspects of a healthy diet is the way in which it allows us to develop a deeper understanding and connection with our bodies. By listening to our hunger and fullness cues and being aware of how different foods make us feel, we open up a whole new level of insight and awareness around nutrition and wellness. This not only helps us make more informed decisions about what and how much to eat, but can also lead to a more joyful and satisfying relationship with food. By prioritizing this deep level of self-awareness and connection, we can achieve long-lasting changes that have a profound impact on our health and wellbeing.

Trying out different ways of eating, such as a plant-based or Mediterranean-style diet, can also be beneficial for health. These dietary patterns emphasize whole, nutrient-dense foods and limit processed and high-fat foods. Additionally, they have been associated with a lower risk of chronic diseases like cardiovascular disease and type 2 diabetes.

Searching for healthy foods can involve looking for nutrient-dense options that provide a variety of vitamins, minerals, and other important nutrients. Foods like fruits, vegetables, whole grains, lean proteins, and healthy fats can help meet nutrient needs while also providing a range of health benefits. It's important to remember that there is no **one-size-fits-all approach to nutrition**, and that the best way of eating is one that meets your individual needs and preferences and is sustainable for the long-term.

I hope that this information has given you a better insight on what foods you are addicted to and the ones that prevent you from being in perfect health. Sometimes just taking them out of your plate just for a short while will show you the inconvenience they cause. To be mindful of our health is the basis of a thriving life.

The saying "you are what you eat" emphasizes the importance of healthy eating habits for overall health and well-being. Research has shown that the type of food we eat can have a significant impact on our physical and mental health, including our risk for chronic diseases like heart disease, diabetes, and cancer. Eating a diet rich in fruits, vegetables, whole grains, lean proteins, and healthy fats can provide the necessary nutrients for good health, while limiting processed and unhealthy foods can help reduce the risk of negative health outcomes. By making informed decisions about what we eat and how we nourish our bodies, we can better support our overall health and well-being.

Treating our bodies as temples of God is the spiritual aspect of nourishing ourselves with wholesome, healthy food. By elevating the act of eating to a sacred practice, we can tap into a level of consciousness and connection that goes far beyond the physical realm. It is through this approach that we can raise our vibrations, making it possible to access higher levels of reality and thrive in this world and beyond. This deep level of reverence for our bodies not only promotes physical health and vitality, but also has the power to transform our entire being, opening up new levels of awareness and spiritual growth. As we treat ourselves with love and respect through the nourishing food we consume, we connect with the divine within and experience a transformative journey towards a more vibrant, joyous life.

Let your food be your medicine

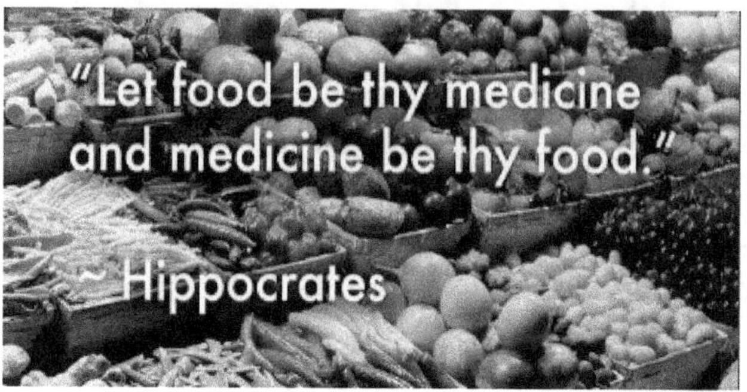

If you have experienced health problems, chronic disease, or sickness, it's important to remember that help is available, and can be found in food. Although it can be more challenging, it is possible to heal from many illnesses by changing the way you eat. Countless individuals have shared their inspiring stories of recovering from cancer, diabetes, chronic fatigue, fibromyalgia, and other health issues by prioritizing nourishing, wholesome foods.

Trusting solely in the medical system may not always lead to optimal health outcomes. The system often does not focus on the cause of the problem but rather on the symptoms with medications. While medication can be beneficial in certain cases, it is important to recognize that it may not always address the root cause of an illness or provide a long-term solution.

The journey towards restored health may not be easy, but with the right mindset and determination, it is possible to achieve a full and vibrant life. Embrace the power of dietary change and discover a new level of physical and spiritual nourishment that can transform your life.

It is possible to live until 100 and beyond. In fact, the number of centenarians (people who have reached the age of 100 or more) is increasing due to advancements in healthcare, nutrition, and lifestyle. According to the United Nations, there were an estimated 316,600 living centenarians worldwide in 2012, and this number is expected to increase substantially in the 21st century. Although genetics can play a role in longevity, healthy lifestyle habits such as a nutritious diet, regular exercise, and stress management can also have a significant impact on our lifespan.

It's important to feel **empowered** and **in charge** of your own life if you want to **thrive** and **enjoy** everything life has to offer. This is especially true today, with all of the resources and opportunities available to us. I encourage you to take a moment to reflect on your goals and aspirations, and to envision where you want to be 10, 20, or 30 years from now. With the right mindset, determination, and a sense of purpose, **anything is possible**. So go ahead, look yourself in the mirror, and take the first step towards a thriving, fulfilling life.

Not a diet but
an eye-opening tool

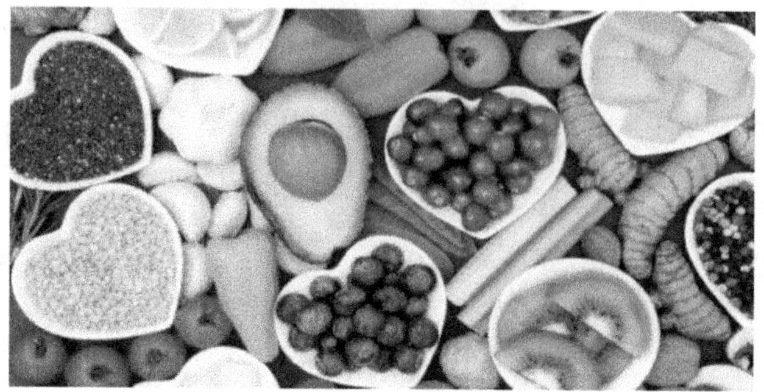

In this book, I want to emphasize that it is not a rigid diet plan that you must strictly follow. I don't claim to have all the knowledge about food, but I have personally incorporated certain elements into my own diet that have proven effective for me. Having struggled with weight and health issues for years, I reached a point where I realized I needed to take control of my eating habits. Surprisingly, I discovered that making simple changes could have a profound impact on my well-being.

Through my own journey, I wanted to share what I've learned about the power of food and how it has transformed my life. My intention is to provide you with valuable information and inspire you to conduct your own research.

By reading this book, I hope it will encourage you to take a moment to reflect on your own health and make informed choices. I understand the challenges that come with changing habits, but I want to assure you that it's never too late to make positive changes and live a vibrant, thriving life.

Your personal nutrition diary

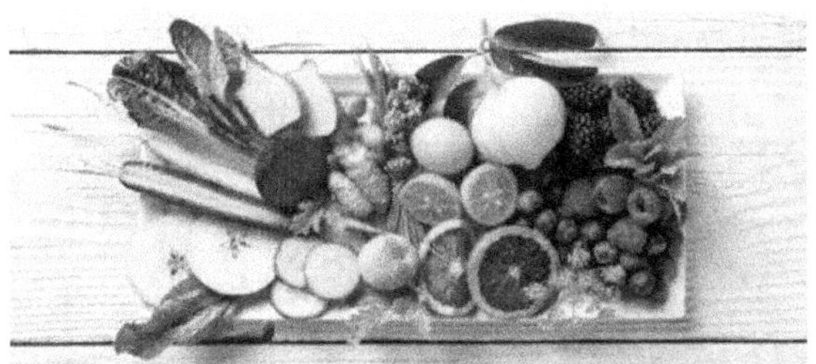

I have put together a little diary to track your progress over the course of 21 days. You can journal your journey and observe the improvements you have noticed.

I encourage you to use this diary to document any symptoms you may face along the way, and put write them as challenges. Whether it's weight loss, bad sleep, digestion problems, or any other issues you encounter, writing them down will help you identify patterns and find ways to overcome them.

You can journal on new habits into your lifestyle. Choose from fasting, juicing, incorporating more raw foods, or simply eliminating sugar, dairy products, or cereals from your diet.

Lastly, I recommend listing the specific foods you are trying to eliminate from your diet. This will help you stay focused and accountable, giving you a clear picture of what you have successfully removed from your daily intake.

This journaling exercise can be repeated every 21 days. Each cycle is an opportunity to introduce something new and track your progress. Embrace this journey with enthusiasm and curiosity, and may this diary serve as a testament to your growth and dedication.

May you flourish and prosper in your life

<table>
<tr><td colspan="4" align="center">Week 1</td></tr>
<tr><td colspan="4" align="center">'True fulfillment comes from embracing challenges and conquering them with courage and determination."</td></tr>
<tr><td colspan="4" align="center">Day 1</td></tr>
<tr><td>Measurement:</td><td colspan="3">Weight</td></tr>
<tr><td>Collar</td><td>Chest</td><td>Waist</td><td>Ankle L   R</td></tr>
<tr><td>Challenges</td><td colspan="3"></td></tr>
<tr><td></td><td colspan="3"></td></tr>
<tr><td>New Habit</td><td colspan="3"></td></tr>
<tr><td></td><td colspan="3"></td></tr>
<tr><td>New foods</td><td colspan="3"></td></tr>
<tr><td></td><td colspan="3"></td></tr>
<tr><td>Food taken out</td><td colspan="3"></td></tr>
<tr><td>Benefits</td><td colspan="3"></td></tr>
<tr><td></td><td colspan="3"></td></tr>
</table>

Day 2

Challenges	
New Habit	
New foods	
Food taken out	
Benefits	

Day 3

Challenges	
New Habit	
New foods	
Food taken out	
Benefits	

Day 4

Challenges	
New Habit	
New foods	
Food taken out	
Benefits	

Day 5

Challenges	
New Habit	
New foods	
Food taken out	
Benefits	

Day 6

Challenges	
New Habit	
New foods	
Food taken out	
Benefits	

Day 7

Challenges	
New Habit	
New foods	
Food taken out	
Benefits	

Week 2

"True growth comes from challenging ourselves to reach new heights,

for it is in discomfort that we discover our limitless potential."

Day 8			
Measurement:	Weight		
Collar	Chest	Waist	Ankle L R
Challenges			
New Habit			
New foods			
Food taken out			
Benefits			

Day 9	
Challenges	
New Habit	
New foods	
Food taken out	
Benefits	

Day 10

Challenges	
New Habit	
New foods	
Food taken out	
Benefits	

Day 11

Challenges	
New Habit	
New foods	
Food taken out	
Benefits	

Day 12

Challenges	
New Habit	
New foods	
Food taken out	
Benefits	

Day 13

Challenges	
New Habit	
New foods	
Food taken out	
Benefits	

Day 14

Challenges	
New Habit	
New foods	
Food taken out	
Benefits	
	0

"Learning is the key that unlocks the door to wisdom, making us wiser with each new lesson we embrace."

Day 15			
Measurement:	Weight		
Collar	Chest	Waist	Ankle L R
Challenges			
New Habit			
New foods			
Food taken out			
Benefits			

Day 16	
Challenges	
New Habit	
New foods	
Food taken out	
Benefits	

Day 17

Challenges	
New Habit	
New foods	
Food taken out	
Benefits	

Day 18

Challenges	
New Habit	
New foods	
Food taken out	
Benefits	

Day 19

Challenges	
New Habit	
New foods	
Food taken out	
Benefits	

Day 20

Challenges	
New Habit	
New foods	
Food taken out	
Benefits	

Day 21

Measurement:	Weight		
Collar	Chest	Waist	Ankle L R
Challenges			
Benefits			

What I have learned from myself and my new eating habits.

Additional notes :